THE COMPLETE AFIB DIET COOKBOOK FOR SENIORS

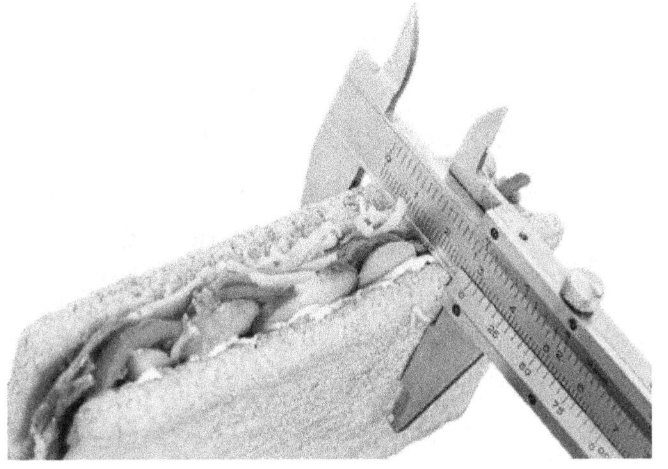

Delicious Recipes for Heart-Healthy Living: Nourishing Your Wellness Journey in the Golden Years

Shannon Christiansen

Table of Contents

INTRODUCTION

Welcome to the AFib Diet Cookbook for Seniors, a culinary journey designed to empower and inspire individuals managing Atrial Fibrillation (AFib) on the path to heart-healthy living. This cookbook is more than just a collection of recipes; it's a compass guiding you towards flavorful meals that nourish your heart and invigorate your well-being.

As we age, the significance of a heart-healthy diet becomes paramount, especially for those navigating the complexities of AFib. This cookbook is crafted with the understanding that delicious meals can be both a source of joy and a powerful tool in the management of cardiovascular health. By embracing nutrient-dense ingredients and mindful cooking practices, we aim to cultivate a positive relationship with food that promotes vitality and longevity.

In these pages, you'll discover a diverse array of recipes carefully curated to suit the tastes and nutritional needs of seniors managing AFib. From wholesome breakfasts to satisfying dinners, delightful snacks to delectable desserts, each recipe is thoughtfully crafted to prioritize

heart health without compromising on flavor.
It's an invitation to savor the goodness of fresh,
whole foods while navigating the unique
considerations of an AFib-friendly diet.

We understand that each individual's journey
with AFib is unique, and dietary choices should
be personalized. Therefore, we encourage you
to embark on this culinary adventure with
curiosity and a willingness to tailor recipes to
your specific preferences and health
requirements. Before making significant
changes to your diet, consult with healthcare
professionals, including cardiologists and
registered dietitians, to ensure your choices
align with your overall wellness plan.

This cookbook is more than just a guide; it's a
companion on your quest for a heart-healthy
lifestyle. Through the recipes within, we hope
to inspire you to embrace the joy of cooking,
the pleasure of savoring nourishing meals, and
the empowerment that comes with actively
contributing to your cardiovascular health.

May this cookbook be a source of delicious
inspiration, encouraging you to relish the
flavors of wholesome ingredients and embark
on a journey towards heart-healthy living,
savoring every moment along the way.

Welcome to a world where nutritious meals become a celebration of life and well-being.

HOW TO USE THIS COOKBOOK

Using a cookbook focused on a heart-healthy AFIB (Atrial Fibrillation) diet for seniors can be a helpful tool for maintaining good cardiovascular health. Here's a guide on how to use the cookbook effectively:

Read the Introduction:

Start by reading the introduction of the cookbook. This section often provides valuable information about the principles of a heart-healthy AFIB diet, key nutrients, and general guidelines.

Consult with a Healthcare Professional:

Before starting any new diet plan, especially if you have a specific health condition like AFIB, it's crucial to consult with your healthcare professional or a registered dietitian. They can provide personalized advice based on your health status and dietary needs.

Review the Recipes:

Browse through the recipes in the cookbook to get an overview of the variety of meals, snacks, and desserts available. Pay attention to the ingredients and nutritional information provided for each recipe.

Create a Meal Plan:

Plan your meals for the week based on the recipes in the cookbook. Consider incorporating a mix of breakfasts, lunches, dinners, and snacks to ensure a balanced and varied diet.

Make a Shopping List:

Once you've decided on your meals, create a shopping list with all the necessary ingredients. This will help you stay organized and ensure you have everything you need when preparing meals.

Follow the Recipes:

When preparing meals, follow the recipes closely. Pay attention to portion sizes, cooking methods, and suggested substitutions if any. The cookbook likely provides clear instructions for each recipe.

Track Your Progress:

Keep a food diary or use a nutrition tracking app to monitor your food intake. This can help you stay on track with your heart-healthy diet and identify any patterns or areas for improvement.

Adapt to Preferences and Dietary Needs:

Feel free to adapt the recipes based on your personal preferences and dietary needs. If you have specific allergies or intolerances, make substitutions as necessary. Remember to keep the overall nutritional balance in mind.

Stay Hydrated:

In addition to meals, don't forget to stay hydrated. Water is crucial for overall health, including heart health. Consider incorporating herbal teas or infused water for variety.

Enjoy in Moderation:

While the recipes are designed to be heart-healthy, it's essential to enjoy meals in moderation. Pay attention to portion sizes and avoid excessive consumption of high-calorie or high-sugar items.

Regular Check-ins:

Periodically check in with your healthcare professional to discuss your diet and its impact on your health. They can provide guidance on any necessary adjustments based on your progress and any changes in your health.

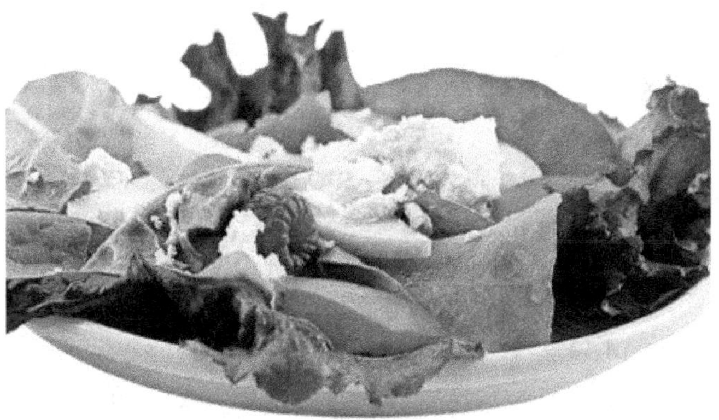

THE IMPORTANCE OF A HEART HEALTHY DIET IN REVERSING ATRIAL FIBRILLATION

Blood Pressure Management:

A heart-healthy diet, rich in fruits, vegetables, and whole grains while low in sodium, can help manage blood pressure. High blood pressure is a common risk factor for AFib, and controlling it can contribute to symptom improvement.

Reducing Inflammation:

Foods with anti-inflammatory properties, such as those rich in antioxidants and omega-3 fatty acids, can help reduce inflammation in the body. Chronic inflammation is associated with cardiovascular diseases, including AFib.

Managing Cholesterol Levels:

A diet focused on healthy fats, such as those found in fish, nuts, and olive oil, can contribute to managing cholesterol levels. Elevated cholesterol is a risk factor for heart disease, and maintaining optimal levels is beneficial for overall heart health.

Weight Management:

Maintaining a healthy weight through a balanced diet is crucial for individuals with AFib. Excess body weight can strain the heart and contribute to the development or worsening of AFib symptoms.

Stabilizing Blood Sugar Levels:

A heart-healthy diet that includes whole grains, lean proteins, and low-glycemic foods can help stabilize blood sugar levels. Blood sugar fluctuations can impact cardiovascular health and potentially contribute to AFib.

Balancing Electrolytes:

Consuming foods rich in potassium and magnesium, such as bananas, leafy greens, and nuts, can help maintain a balance of electrolytes. This is important for heart function and may contribute to AFib symptom management.

Minimizing Triggers:

Certain dietary components, such as excessive caffeine or alcohol, may act as triggers for AFib episodes. A heart-healthy diet can help minimize these triggers and reduce the likelihood of symptom exacerbation.

Optimizing Nutrient Intake:

A nutrient-dense diet ensures the intake of essential vitamins and minerals necessary for overall health. Nutritional deficiencies can impact heart function, and maintaining optimal nutrient levels is important for individuals with AFib.

Improving Cardiovascular Health:

A heart-healthy diet contributes to overall cardiovascular well-being. It supports healthy blood vessels, improves circulation, and enhances the heart's ability to function efficiently.

Enhancing Overall Well-Being:

Beyond specific considerations for AFib, a heart-healthy diet promotes overall well-being. It can increase energy levels, support immune function, and contribute to a higher quality of life.

While dietary changes are an important aspect of AFib management, it's crucial to approach them as part of a comprehensive care plan. Individuals with AFib should work closely with healthcare professionals, including cardiologists and registered dietitians, to develop a personalized approach that considers their unique health status and needs. Lifestyle modifications, including dietary changes, are typically one component of a multifaceted approach to managing AFib.

FOOD TO AVOID

For individuals with Atrial Fibrillation (AFib), certain dietary modifications can contribute to better heart health and overall well-being. While it's essential to focus on a heart-healthy diet, it's equally important to be mindful of foods that may potentially trigger or exacerbate AFib symptoms. Here are some foods to consider limiting or avoiding in an AFib diet for seniors:

Caffeine:

Excessive caffeine intake, found in coffee, tea, energy drinks, and certain sodas, may stimulate the heart and potentially contribute to irregular heart rhythms. It's advisable to moderate caffeine consumption.

Alcohol:

Alcohol can be a trigger for AFib in some individuals. Limiting alcohol intake, or avoiding it altogether, can be beneficial. If consumed, it should be in moderation, following the recommendations of healthcare professionals.

High-Sodium Foods:

Excessive sodium intake can contribute to high blood pressure, which is a risk factor for AFib. Avoid processed foods, canned soups, and high-sodium snacks. Opt for fresh, whole foods and season meals with herbs and spices instead of salt.

Processed and Fried Foods:

Processed and fried foods are often high in unhealthy fats and may contribute to inflammation and heart issues. Choose heart-healthy cooking methods like grilling, baking, or steaming, and focus on whole, nutrient-dense foods.

Certain Types of Fish:

Some types of fish, such as mackerel and tuna, are high in mercury. Excessive mercury intake may be associated with heart rhythm issues. Choose low-mercury fish like salmon, trout, and sardines.

Fatty Cuts of Meat:

High-fat meats, especially those with saturated fats, can contribute to high cholesterol and heart issues. Choose lean cuts of meat, poultry without skin, and incorporate plant-based protein sources like beans and legumes.

Artificial Sweeteners:

Some individuals may be sensitive to artificial sweeteners, and they could potentially trigger AFib symptoms. Consider natural sweeteners in moderation, such as honey or maple syrup.

High-Glycemic Foods:

Foods with a high glycemic index can cause rapid spikes in blood sugar levels, potentially impacting heart health. Choose whole grains, legumes, and fruits with lower glycemic index values.

Spicy Foods:

Spicy foods may trigger symptoms in some individuals. Pay attention to personal tolerance levels and limit the intake of extremely spicy foods.

High-Cholesterol Foods:

Foods high in cholesterol, such as organ meats and certain shellfish, may contribute to elevated cholesterol levels. Choose lean proteins and plant-based sources of protein.

Approved dietary cardiologist guidelines for AFIB

Heart-Healthy Diet:

Emphasize a heart-healthy diet, which typically includes a variety of fruits, vegetables, whole grains, lean proteins, and healthy fats. Such a diet provides essential nutrients, fiber, and antioxidants.

Limit Sodium Intake:

Reduce sodium intake to help manage blood pressure. This involves minimizing the consumption of processed and packaged foods, as they often contain high levels of sodium.

Moderate Caffeine Intake:

While there's no strict ban on caffeine, moderate its intake. Excessive caffeine consumption may contribute to irregular heart rhythms in some individuals. Individual tolerance levels can vary.

Moderate Alcohol Consumption:

If alcohol is consumed, it's generally advised to do so in moderation. Excessive alcohol intake can contribute to AFib in some cases. Moderation is typically defined as up to one drink per day for women and up to two drinks per day for men.

Maintain a Healthy Weight:

Achieve and maintain a healthy weight to reduce the risk of cardiovascular issues. Weight management often involves a combination of a balanced diet and regular physical activity.

Limit Processed Foods and Trans Fats:

Minimize the intake of processed and fried foods, as well as foods high in trans fats. Focus on whole, nutrient-dense foods to support overall heart health.

Omega-3 Fatty Acids:

Include sources of omega-3 fatty acids in the diet, such as fatty fish (e.g., salmon, mackerel), flaxseeds, chia seeds, and walnuts. Omega-3s are associated with heart health.

Regular Physical Activity:

Engage in regular physical activity as part of a heart-healthy lifestyle. Exercise is essential for overall cardiovascular health and may contribute to better AFib management.

Stay Hydrated:

Maintain proper hydration by drinking an adequate amount of water. Dehydration can sometimes contribute to AFib episodes.

Individualized Approach:

Recognize that dietary needs may vary among individuals. An individualized approach that takes into account overall health, existing medical conditions, and personal preferences is crucial.

BREAKFAST RECIPES

Oatmeal with Berries and Almonds:

- Ingredients: 1/2 cup old-fashioned oats, 1 cup mixed berries, 1 tablespoon chopped almonds.
- Preparation: Cook oats with water, top with berries and almonds.
- Prep Time: 10 minutes.
- Calories: Approximately 250.
- Nutritional Information: High in fiber, antioxidants, and heart-healthy fats.

Greek Yogurt Parfait:

- Ingredients: 1 cup low-fat Greek yogurt, 1/2 cup granola, 1/2 cup fresh fruit (e.g., strawberries or blueberries).
- Preparation: Layer yogurt, granola, and fruit in a glass.
- Prep Time: 5 minutes.
- Calories: Around 300.
- Nutritional Information: Rich in protein, probiotics, and vitamins.

Spinach and Feta Egg Muffins:

- Ingredients: 4 eggs, 1 cup fresh spinach, 1/4 cup feta cheese.
- Preparation: Whisk eggs, mix with spinach and feta, bake in muffin tin.
- Prep Time: 20 minutes.
- Calories: Approximately 200.
- Nutritional Information: High in protein, vitamins, and minerals.

Whole Wheat Pancakes with Banana:

- Ingredients: 1 cup whole wheat flour, 1 cup milk, 1 egg, 1 mashed banana.
- Preparation: Mix ingredients, cook on a griddle, top with sliced bananas.
- Prep Time: 15 minutes.
- Calories: Around 250.
- Nutritional Information: Good source of fiber, potassium, and whole grains.

Chia Seed Pudding:

- Ingredients: 3 tablespoons chia seeds, 1 cup almond milk, 1/2 teaspoon vanilla extract.

- Preparation: Mix ingredients, refrigerate overnight, top with fresh fruit.
- Prep Time: 5 minutes (plus overnight soaking).
- Calories: Approximately 180.
- Nutritional Information: Rich in omega-3 fatty acids, fiber, and calcium.

Smoothie Bowl with Kale and Berry Blend:

- Ingredients: 1 cup kale, 1/2 cup mixed berries, 1/2 banana, 1/2 cup almond milk.
- Preparation: Blend ingredients, top with granola and sliced almonds.
- Prep Time: 10 minutes.
- Calories: Around 220.
- Nutritional Information: Packed with vitamins, antioxidants, and fiber.

Avocado Toast with Poached Egg:

- Ingredients: 1 slice whole grain bread, 1/2 avocado, 1 poached egg.
- Preparation: Toast bread, spread avocado, top with poached egg.
- Prep Time: 15 minutes.
- Calories: Approximately 300.

- Nutritional Information: Rich in heart-healthy fats and protein.

Quinoa Breakfast Bowl:

- Ingredients: 1/2 cup cooked quinoa, 1/4 cup chopped nuts, 1/2 cup diced fruit (e.g., mango or pineapple).
- Preparation: Mix ingredients, drizzle with honey.
- Prep Time: 15 minutes.
- Calories: Around 280.
- Nutritional Information: High in protein, fiber, and vitamins.

Salmon and Cream Cheese Bagel:

- Ingredients: 1 whole grain bagel, 2 ounces smoked salmon, 2 tablespoons low-fat cream cheese, cucumber slices.
- Preparation: Toast bagel, spread cream cheese, top with salmon and cucumber.
- Prep Time: 10 minutes.
- Calories: Approximately 350.
- Nutritional Information: Rich in omega-3 fatty acids, protein, and calcium.

Fruit and Nut Yogurt Bowl:

- Ingredients: 1 cup low-fat yogurt, 1/2 cup mixed nuts, 1/2 cup diced mixed fruit.
- Preparation: Combine ingredients in a bowl.
- Prep Time: 5 minutes.
- Calories: Around 280.
- Nutritional Information: High in protein, fiber, and essential nutrients.

LUNCH RECIPES

Grilled Salmon Salad:

- Ingredients: 4 ounces grilled salmon, mixed salad greens, cherry tomatoes, cucumber slices.
- Preparation: Toss ingredients together, drizzle with olive oil and lemon.
- Prep Time: 15 minutes.
- Calories: Approximately 350.
- Nutritional Information: Rich in omega-3 fatty acids, antioxidants, and vitamins.

Quinoa and Vegetable Stir-Fry:

- Ingredients: 1/2 cup cooked quinoa, assorted stir-fry vegetables, tofu or lean chicken.
- Preparation: Stir-fry vegetables and protein, mix with quinoa.
- Prep Time: 20 minutes.
- Calories: Around 300.
- Nutritional Information: High in fiber, protein, and essential nutrients.

Turkey and Avocado Wrap:

- Ingredients: Whole grain wrap, 3 ounces sliced turkey breast, 1/4 avocado, lettuce, tomato.
- Preparation: Assemble ingredients in the wrap.
- Prep Time: 10 minutes.
- Calories: Approximately 300.
- Nutritional Information: Lean protein, heart-healthy fats, and fiber.

Mediterranean Chickpea Salad:

- Ingredients: Canned chickpeas, cherry tomatoes, cucumber, feta cheese, olives.
- Preparation: Combine ingredients, drizzle with olive oil and balsamic vinegar.
- Prep Time: 15 minutes.
- Calories: Around 250.
- Nutritional Information: High in fiber, plant-based protein, and antioxidants.

Spinach and Lentil Soup:

- Ingredients: Spinach, lentils, carrots, celery, low-sodium vegetable broth.
- Preparation: Simmer ingredients until lentils are tender.

- Prep Time: 30 minutes.
- Calories: Approximately 200.
- Nutritional Information: Rich in fiber, iron, and vitamins.

Chicken and Vegetable Skewers:

- Ingredients: Chicken breast, bell peppers, cherry tomatoes, zucchini.
- Preparation: Thread ingredients onto skewers, grill until chicken is cooked.
- Prep Time: 25 minutes.
- Calories: Around 280.
- Nutritional Information: Lean protein, vitamins, and antioxidants.

Whole Grain Pasta with Pesto and Vegetables:

- Ingredients: Whole grain pasta, homemade basil pesto, cherry tomatoes, broccoli.
- Preparation: Cook pasta, toss with pesto and vegetables.
- Prep Time: 20 minutes.
- Calories: Approximately 320.
- Nutritional Information: Whole grains, healthy fats, and vitamins.

Salmon and Vegetable Quiche:

- Ingredients: Whole wheat pie crust, eggs, salmon, spinach, bell peppers.
- Preparation: Whisk eggs, mix with other ingredients, bake.
- Prep Time: 40 minutes.
- Calories: Around 350.
- Nutritional Information: Protein, omega-3 fatty acids, and vegetables.

Black Bean and Vegetable Burrito Bowl:

- Ingredients: Brown rice, black beans, corn, salsa, avocado.
- Preparation: Assemble ingredients in a bowl.
- Prep Time: 15 minutes.
- Calories: Approximately 300.
- Nutritional Information: High in fiber, plant-based protein, and essential nutrients.

Shrimp and Quinoa Stuffed Bell Peppers:

- Ingredients: Bell peppers, shrimp, quinoa, tomatoes, onions.
- Preparation: Cook quinoa, mix with other ingredients, stuff peppers, bake.
- Prep Time: 30 minutes.

- Calories: Around 320.
- Nutritional Information: Protein, fiber, and vitamins.

DINNER RECIPES

Baked Lemon Herb Chicken:

- Ingredients: Chicken breast, lemon juice, garlic, rosemary, thyme.
- Preparation: Marinate chicken, bake until fully cooked.
- Prep Time: 30 minutes.
- Calories: Approximately 300.
- Nutritional Information: High in lean protein, low in saturated fat.

Vegetable and Lentil Curry:

- Ingredients: Lentils, mixed vegetables, tomatoes, curry spices.
- Preparation: Cook lentils, sauté vegetables, simmer with spices.
- Prep Time: 40 minutes.
- Calories: Around 250.
- Nutritional Information: Rich in fiber, plant-based protein, and antioxidants.

Salmon and Asparagus Foil Packets:

- Ingredients: Salmon fillet, asparagus, lemon, dill.
- Preparation: Place ingredients in foil packets, bake or grill.
- Prep Time: 25 minutes.
- Calories: Approximately 320.
- Nutritional Information: Omega-3 fatty acids, vitamins, and minerals.

Quinoa-Stuffed Bell Peppers

- Ingredients: Quinoa, black beans, corn, tomatoes, spices.
- Preparation: Cook quinoa, mix with other ingredients, stuff peppers, bake.
- Prep Time: 40 minutes.
- Calories: Around 300.
- Nutritional Information: High in fiber, plant-based protein, and essential nutrients.

Turkey and Vegetable Stir-Fry:

- Ingredients: Ground turkey, broccoli, bell peppers, ginger, soy sauce.

- Preparation: Stir-fry ingredients, add soy sauce and spices.
- Prep Time: 20 minutes.
- Calories: Approximately 280.
- Nutritional Information: Lean protein, vegetables, low in sodium.

Baked Cod with Tomato and Olive Salsa:

- Ingredients: Cod fillet, tomatoes, olives, garlic, basil.
- Preparation: Mix salsa ingredients, spoon over cod, bake.
- Prep Time: 25 minutes.
- Calories: Around 250.
- Nutritional Information: Lean protein, antioxidants, and healthy fats.

Chickpea and Vegetable Curry:

- Ingredients: Chickpeas, cauliflower, spinach, tomatoes, curry spices.
- Preparation: Cook chickpeas, sauté vegetables, simmer with spices.
- Prep Time: 35 minutes.
- Calories: Approximately 270.
- Nutritional Information: Plant-based protein, fiber, and vitamins.

Grilled Vegetable and Quinoa Salad:

- Ingredients: Quinoa, mixed grilled vegetables, feta cheese, balsamic vinaigrette.
- Preparation: Cook quinoa, toss with grilled veggies, top with feta and dressing.
- Prep Time: 30 minutes.
- Calories: Around 320.
- Nutritional Information: High in fiber, antioxidants, and vitamins.

Chicken and Vegetable Skewers with Brown Rice:

- Ingredients: Chicken breast, bell peppers, onions, cherry tomatoes, brown rice.
- Preparation: Thread ingredients onto skewers, grill, serve over cooked brown rice.
- Prep Time: 35 minutes.
- Calories: Approximately 330.
- Nutritional Information: Lean protein, fiber, and essential nutrients.

Sweet Potato and Black Bean Chili:

- Ingredients: Sweet potatoes, black beans, tomatoes, chili spices.
- Preparation: Cook sweet potatoes, add black beans, tomatoes, and spices, simmer.
- Prep Time: 40 minutes.
- Calories: Around 290.
- Nutritional Information: High in fiber, plant-based protein, and vitamins.

SWEET DESSERTS

Berry Parfait:

- Ingredients: Mixed berries (strawberries, blueberries, raspberries), low-fat Greek yogurt, granola.
- Preparation: Layer berries, yogurt, and granola in a glass.
- Prep Time: 10 minutes.
- Calories: Approximately 200.
- Nutritional Information: High in antioxidants, fiber, and probiotics.

Dark Chocolate-Dipped Strawberries:

- Ingredients: Fresh strawberries, dark chocolate (70% cocoa or higher).
- Preparation: Melt dark chocolate, dip strawberries, let them cool.
- Prep Time: 20 minutes.
- Calories: Around 150.
- Nutritional Information: Rich in antioxidants and heart-healthy flavonoids.

Baked Apples with Cinnamon and Walnuts:

- Ingredients: Apples, cinnamon, chopped walnuts, a drizzle of honey.
- Preparation: Core apples, fill with cinnamon and walnuts, bake until tender.
- Prep Time: 30 minutes.
- Calories: Approximately 180.
- Nutritional Information: High in fiber, vitamins, and healthy fats.

Chia Seed Pudding with Mango:

- Ingredients: Chia seeds, almond milk, vanilla extract, diced mango.
- Preparation: Mix chia seeds with almond milk and vanilla, refrigerate, top with mango.
- Prep Time: 10 minutes (plus chilling).
- Calories: Around 220.
- Nutritional Information: Omega-3 fatty acids, fiber, and vitamins.

Frozen Banana Bites:

- Ingredients: Sliced bananas, natural peanut butter, dark chocolate.
- Preparation: Spread peanut butter between banana slices, dip in melted dark chocolate, freeze.

- Prep Time: 15 minutes (plus freezing).
- Calories: Approximately 160.
- Nutritional Information: Potassium, healthy fats, and antioxidants.

Yogurt and Berry Popsicles:

- Ingredients: Low-fat yogurt, mixed berries, a touch of honey.
- Preparation: Blend yogurt, berries, and honey, pour into popsicle molds, freeze.
- Prep Time: 15 minutes (plus freezing).
- Calories: Around 120.
- Nutritional Information: Probiotics, antioxidants, and vitamins.

Cinnamon Baked Pears:

- Ingredients: Pears, cinnamon, a sprinkle of chopped almonds.
- Preparation: Slice pears, sprinkle with cinnamon, bake, top with almonds.
- Prep Time: 25 minutes.
- Calories: Approximately 160.
- Nutritional Information: High in fiber, vitamins, and healthy fats.

Coconut and Mango Sorbet:

- Ingredients: Frozen mango chunks, coconut milk, a touch of lime juice.
- Preparation: Blend mango, coconut milk, and lime juice until smooth, freeze.
- Prep Time: 10 minutes (plus freezing).
- Calories: Around 180.
- Nutritional Information: Vitamins, healthy fats, and a natural sweetness.

Almond and Berry Crisp:

- Ingredients: Mixed berries, oats, almond flour, chopped almonds.
- Preparation: Mix berries with a sprinkle of almond flour, top with a mixture of oats and chopped almonds, bake.
- Prep Time: 35 minutes.
- Calories: Approximately 210.
- Nutritional Information: Fiber, antioxidants, and healthy fats.

Peach and Ginger Smoothie Bowl:

- Ingredients: Frozen peaches, Greek yogurt, fresh ginger, a drizzle of honey.

- Preparation: Blend peaches, yogurt, and ginger until smooth, pour into a bowl, drizzle with honey.
- Prep Time: 10 minutes.
- Calories: Around 230.
- Nutritional Information: Probiotics, vitamins, and anti-inflammatory properties.

SNACKS AND APPETIZERS

Hummus and Veggie Platter:

- Ingredients: Hummus, carrot sticks, cucumber slices, cherry tomatoes.
- Preparation: Arrange veggies around a bowl of hummus for dipping.
- Prep Time: 10 minutes.
- Calories: Around 150.
- Nutritional Information: Fiber, vitamins, and healthy fats.

Guacamole with Whole Grain Pita Chips:

- Ingredients: Avocado, tomato, onion, lime, whole grain pita.
- Preparation: Mash avocado, mix with diced veggies, serve with baked pita chips.
- Prep Time: 15 minutes.
- Calories: Approximately 180.
- Nutritional Information: Healthy fats, fiber, and vitamins.

Greek Yogurt and Berry Parfait:

- Ingredients: Low-fat Greek yogurt, mixed berries, a sprinkle of granola.
- Preparation: Layer yogurt, berries, and granola in a glass.
- Prep Time: 10 minutes.
- Calories: Around 200.
- Nutritional Information: Protein, probiotics, antioxidants.

Cucumber and Smoked Salmon Bites:

- Ingredients: Cucumber slices, smoked salmon, dill.
- Preparation: Top cucumber slices with smoked salmon, garnish with dill.
- Prep Time: 15 minutes.
- Calories: Approximately 120.
- Nutritional Information: Omega-3 fatty acids, protein, and vitamins.

Edamame and Sea Salt:

- Ingredients: Edamame, sea salt.
- Preparation: Steam edamame, sprinkle with sea salt.
- Prep Time: 5 minutes.
- Calories: Around 100.
- Nutritional Information: Protein, fiber, and essential minerals.

Baked Sweet Potato Fries:

- Ingredients: Sweet potatoes, olive oil, rosemary.
- Preparation: Cut sweet potatoes into fries, toss with olive oil and rosemary, bake.
- Prep Time: 30 minutes.
- Calories: Approximately 150.
- Nutritional Information: Fiber, vitamins, and antioxidants.

Whole Grain Crackers with Cottage Cheese and Berries:

- Ingredients: Whole grain crackers, low-fat cottage cheese, mixed berries.
- Preparation: Spread cottage cheese on crackers, top with berries.
- Prep Time: 10 minutes.
- Calories: Around 180.
- Nutritional Information: Protein, fiber, and antioxidants.

Roasted Chickpeas:

- Ingredients: Canned chickpeas, olive oil, cumin, paprika.
- Preparation: Toss chickpeas with olive oil and spices, roast until crunchy.

- Prep Time: 40 minutes.
- Calories: Approximately 150.
- Nutritional Information: Protein, fiber, and minerals.

Caprese Salad Skewers:

- Ingredients: Cherry tomatoes, fresh mozzarella balls, basil leaves, balsamic glaze.
- Preparation: Thread tomatoes, mozzarella, and basil onto skewers, drizzle with balsamic glaze.
- Prep Time: 15 minutes.
- Calories: Around 160.
- Nutritional Information: Calcium, antioxidants, and healthy fats.

Almond Butter and Banana Slices on Whole Wheat Toast:

- Ingredients: Whole wheat bread, almond butter, banana slices.
- Preparation: Toast bread, spread almond butter, top with banana slices.
- Prep Time: 10 minutes.
- Calories: Approximately 220.
- Nutritional Information: Healthy fats, potassium, and fiber.

SMOOTHIES

Berry Blast Smoothie:

- Ingredients: Mixed berries (strawberries, blueberries, raspberries), low-fat yogurt, almond milk, chia seeds.
- Preparation: Blend berries, yogurt, almond milk, and chia seeds until smooth.
- Prep Time: 5 minutes.
- Calories: Around 200.
- Nutritional Information: Antioxidants, probiotics, omega-3 fatty acids.

Green Power Smoothie:

- Ingredients: Spinach, kale, banana, Greek yogurt, coconut water.
- Preparation: Blend spinach, kale, banana, yogurt, and coconut water until smooth.
- Prep Time: 7 minutes.
- Calories: Approximately 180.
- Nutritional Information: Fiber, vitamins, and probiotics.

Tropical Paradise Smoothie:

- Ingredients: Pineapple, mango, Greek yogurt, orange juice, ice.
- Preparation: Blend pineapple, mango, yogurt, orange juice, and ice until smooth.
- Prep Time: 5 minutes.
- Calories: Around 220.
- Nutritional Information: Vitamin C, probiotics, and antioxidants.

Banana Almond Butter Smoothie:

- Ingredients: Banana, almond butter, low-fat milk, flaxseeds.
- Preparation: Blend banana, almond butter, milk, and flaxseeds until creamy.
- Prep Time: 5 minutes.
- Calories: Approximately 250.
- Nutritional Information: Potassium, healthy fats, and fiber.

Avocado and Spinach Smoothie:

- Ingredients: Avocado, spinach, cucumber, lemon juice, almond milk.
- Preparation: Blend avocado, spinach, cucumber, lemon juice, and almond milk until smooth.
- Prep Time: 7 minutes.
- Calories: Around 230.

- Nutritional Information: Healthy fats, vitamins, and antioxidants.

Peachy Keen Smoothie:

- Ingredients: Peaches, low-fat yogurt, almond milk, a touch of honey.
- Preparation: Blend peaches, yogurt, almond milk, and honey until well combined.
- Prep Time: 6 minutes.
- Calories: Approximately 190.
- Nutritional Information: Vitamins, probiotics, and natural sweetness.

Cocoa Banana Smoothie:

- Ingredients: Banana, unsweetened cocoa powder, low-fat milk, Greek yogurt.
- Preparation: Blend banana, cocoa powder, milk, and yogurt until smooth.
- Prep Time: 5 minutes.
- Calories: Around 210.
- Nutritional Information: Potassium, calcium, and antioxidants.

Cherry Almond Smoothie:

- Ingredients: Cherries, almond milk, low-fat yogurt, ground flaxseeds.

- Preparation: Blend cherries, almond milk, yogurt, and flaxseeds until creamy.
- Prep Time: 6 minutes.
- Calories: Approximately 240.
- Nutritional Information: Antioxidants, probiotics, and healthy fats.

Minty Pineapple Kale Smoothie:

- Ingredients: Pineapple, kale, mint leaves, low-fat yogurt, coconut water.
- Preparation: Blend pineapple, kale, mint, yogurt, and coconut water until smooth.
- Prep Time: 7 minutes.
- Calories: Around 200.
- Nutritional Information: Vitamins, probiotics, and antioxidants.

Strawberry Banana Protein Smoothie:

- Ingredients: Strawberries, banana, protein powder, low-fat milk.
- Preparation: Blend strawberries, banana, protein powder, and milk until well combined.
- Prep Time: 5 minutes.

- Calories: Approximately 250.
- Nutritional Information: Protein, vitamins, and potassium.

BONUS :7DAY MEAL PLAN

Day 1:

Breakfast - Berry Yogurt Parfait:
- Ingredients: Low-fat Greek yogurt, mixed berries (strawberries, blueberries, raspberries), granola.
- Preparation: Layer yogurt, berries, and granola in a glass.
- Prep Time: 10 minutes.
- Calories: Approximately 250.
- Nutritional Information: High in antioxidants, fiber, and probiotics.

Lunch - Grilled Chicken Salad:
- Ingredients: Grilled chicken breast, mixed salad greens, cherry tomatoes, cucumber, balsamic vinaigrette.
- Preparation: Toss salad ingredients together, drizzle with vinaigrette.
- Prep Time: 20 minutes.

- Calories: Around 300.
- Nutritional Information: Lean protein, vitamins, and fiber.

Dinner - Baked Salmon with Quinoa:

- Ingredients: Salmon fillet, quinoa, lemon, olive oil, steamed broccoli.
- Preparation: Season salmon, bake, serve over cooked quinoa with a side of steamed broccoli.
- Prep Time: 30 minutes.
- Calories: Approximately 400.
- Nutritional Information: Omega-3 fatty acids, protein, and fiber.

Snack - Greek Yogurt with Almonds:

- Ingredients: Low-fat Greek yogurt, almonds.
- Preparation: Top yogurt with almonds.
- Prep Time: 5 minutes.
- Calories: Around 150.
- Nutritional Information: Protein, healthy fats, and vitamins.

Day 2:

Breakfast - Oatmeal with Fresh Fruit:

- Ingredients: Rolled oats, almond milk, banana slices, chia seeds.
- Preparation: Cook oats with almond milk, top with banana slices and chia seeds.
- Prep Time: 15 minutes.
- Calories: Approximately 280.
- Nutritional Information: Fiber, potassium, and omega-3 fatty acids.

Lunch - Quinoa and Vegetable Stir-Fry:
- Ingredients: Quinoa, mixed stir-fry vegetables (bell peppers, broccoli, carrots), tofu, low-sodium soy sauce.
- Preparation: Cook quinoa, stir-fry vegetables and tofu with soy sauce.
- Prep Time: 25 minutes.
- Calories: Around 350.
- Nutritional Information: Protein, fiber, and antioxidants.

Dinner - Turkey and Vegetable Skewers:
- Ingredients: Turkey breast, bell peppers, cherry tomatoes, zucchini, olive oil.
- Preparation: Thread turkey and vegetables onto skewers, grill or bake.
- Prep Time: 30 minutes.
- Calories: Approximately 380.

- Nutritional Information: Lean protein, vitamins, and healthy fats.

Snack - Apple Slices with Peanut Butter:
- Ingredients: Apple slices, natural peanut butter.
- Preparation: Spread peanut butter on apple slices.
- Prep Time: 5 minutes.
- Calories: Around 200.
- Nutritional Information: Fiber, healthy fats, and protein.

Day 3:

Breakfast - Spinach and Feta Omelette:
- Ingredients: Eggs, spinach, feta cheese, tomatoes, olive oil.
- Preparation: Whisk eggs, sauté vegetables, pour eggs over, cook, fold, and add feta.
- Prep Time: 15 minutes.
- Calories: Approximately 300.
- Nutritional Information: Protein, vitamins, and healthy fats.

Lunch - Lentil and Vegetable Soup:
- Ingredients: Lentils, carrots, celery, onions, low-sodium vegetable broth.

- Preparation: Cook lentils and vegetables in broth until tender.
- Prep Time: 30 minutes.
- Calories: Around 250.
- Nutritional Information: Fiber, protein, and vitamins.

Dinner - Baked Chicken with Sweet Potato Mash:
- Ingredients: Chicken thighs, sweet potatoes, garlic, rosemary, olive oil.
- Preparation: Season chicken, bake, serve with mashed sweet potatoes.
- Prep Time: 40 minutes.
- Calories: Approximately 400.
- Nutritional Information: Lean protein, beta-carotene, and fiber.

Snack - Mixed Berries Smoothie:
- Ingredients: Mixed berries, low-fat yogurt, almond milk.
- Preparation: Blend berries, yogurt, and almond milk until smooth.
- Prep Time: 10 minutes.
- Calories: Around 180.
- Nutritional Information: Antioxidants, probiotics, and vitamins.

Breakfast - Chia Seed Pudding:

- Ingredients: Chia seeds, almond milk, vanilla extract, mixed berries.
- Preparation: Mix chia seeds with almond milk and vanilla, refrigerate overnight, top with berries.
- Prep Time: 5 minutes (plus overnight soaking).
- Calories: Around 270.
- Nutritional Information: Omega-3 fatty acids, fiber, and antioxidants.

Lunch - Quinoa Salad with Avocado and Chickpeas:

- Ingredients: Quinoa, cherry tomatoes, cucumber, avocado, chickpeas, lemon vinaigrette.
- Preparation: Cook quinoa, toss with vegetables, chickpeas, and lemon vinaigrette.
- Prep Time: 20 minutes.
- Calories: Approximately 320.
- Nutritional Information: Protein, fiber, and healthy fats.

Dinner - Shrimp Stir-Fry with Brown Rice:

- Ingredients: Shrimp, mixed stir-fry vegetables (snap peas, bell peppers, carrots), brown rice, soy sauce.
- Preparation: Stir-fry shrimp and vegetables, serve over cooked brown rice.
- Prep Time: 25 minutes.
- Calories: Around 380.
- Nutritional Information: Protein, fiber, and essential minerals.

Snack - Yogurt and Fruit Bowl:
- Ingredients: Low-fat yogurt, kiwi slices, pomegranate seeds.
- Preparation: Arrange yogurt in a bowl, top with kiwi slices and pomegranate seeds.
- Prep Time: 5 minutes.
- Calories: Approximately 150.
- Nutritional Information: Probiotics, vitamins, and antioxidants.

Day 5:

Breakfast - Banana Walnut Smoothie:
- Ingredients: Banana, walnuts, low-fat milk, plain yogurt.
- Preparation: Blend banana, walnuts, milk, and yogurt until smooth.
- Prep Time: 7 minutes.
- Calories: Around 250.

- Nutritional Information: Potassium, omega-3 fatty acids, and protein.

Lunch - Caprese Quinoa Bowl:
- Ingredients: Quinoa, cherry tomatoes, fresh mozzarella, basil, balsamic glaze.
- Preparation: Combine cooked quinoa with tomatoes, mozzarella, and basil. Drizzle with balsamic glaze.
- Prep Time: 15 minutes.
- Calories: Approximately 300.
- Nutritional Information: Protein, calcium, and antioxidants.

Dinner - Baked Cod with Lemon Herb Sauce:
- Ingredients: Cod fillets, lemon, garlic, thyme, olive oil.
- Preparation: Season cod, bake with lemon and herbs, serve with steamed green beans.
- Prep Time: 30 minutes.
- Calories: Around 350.
- Nutritional Information: Omega-3 fatty acids, protein, and vitamins.

Snack - Mango Salsa with Whole Grain Crackers:
- Ingredients: Diced mango, red onion, cilantro, lime juice, whole grain crackers.

- Preparation: Mix mango, onion, cilantro, and lime juice. Serve with whole grain crackers.
- Prep Time: 10 minutes.
- Calories: Approximately 180.
- Nutritional Information: Fiber, vitamins, and antioxidants.

Day 6:

Breakfast - Spinach and Mushroom Frittata:
- Ingredients: Eggs, spinach, mushrooms, onion, low-fat cheese.
- Preparation: Sauté vegetables, pour whisked eggs over, cook until set, sprinkle with cheese.
- Prep Time: 20 minutes.
- Calories: Approximately 280.
- Nutritional Information: Protein, vitamins, and minerals.

Lunch - Chickpea Salad with Feta:
- Ingredients: Chickpeas, cherry tomatoes, cucumber, red onion, feta cheese, olive oil.
- Preparation: Combine chickpeas, vegetables, and feta. Drizzle with olive oil.
- Prep Time: 15 minutes.
- Calories: Around 320.

- Nutritional Information: Protein, fiber, and healthy fats.

Dinner - Turkey and Vegetable Stir-Fry with Brown Rice:
- Ingredients: Ground turkey, mixed stir-fry vegetables (broccoli, snap peas, carrots), brown rice, low-sodium soy sauce.
- Preparation: Stir-fry turkey and vegetables, serve over cooked brown rice.
- Prep Time: 25 minutes.
- Calories: Approximately 380.
- Nutritional Information: Lean protein, fiber, and essential minerals.

Snack - Hummus and Vegetable Sticks:
- Ingredients: Hummus, carrot sticks, cucumber slices, bell pepper strips.
- Preparation: Dip vegetable sticks into hummus.
- Prep Time: 10 minutes.
- Calories: Around 150.
- Nutritional Information: Protein, fiber, and vitamins.

Day 7:

Breakfast - Blueberry Almond Smoothie Bowl:

- Ingredients: Frozen blueberries, almond milk, banana, almonds, granola.
- Preparation: Blend blueberries, banana, and almond milk. Top with almonds and granola.
- Prep Time: 10 minutes.
- Calories: Approximately 270.
- Nutritional Information: Antioxidants, healthy fats, and fiber.

Lunch - Lentil and Spinach Stuffed Bell Peppers:

- Ingredients: Lentils, spinach, bell peppers, tomatoes, garlic, Italian herbs.
- Preparation: Cook lentils and spinach, stuff bell peppers, bake until tender.
- Prep Time: 30 minutes.
- Calories: Around 300.
- Nutritional Information: Protein, fiber, and vitamins.

Dinner - Grilled Vegetable and Quinoa Bowl:

- Ingredients: Quinoa, grilled vegetables (zucchini, eggplant, bell peppers), lemon tahini dressing.

- Preparation: Cook quinoa, grill vegetables, toss with lemon tahini dressing.
- Prep Time: 25 minutes.
- Calories: Approximately 350.
- Nutritional Information: Protein, fiber, and healthy fats.

Snack - Cottage Cheese with Pineapple:
- Ingredients: Low-fat cottage cheese, pineapple chunks.
- Preparation: Combine cottage cheese with pineapple.
- Prep Time: 5 minutes.
- Calories: Around 180.
- Nutritional Information: Protein, vitamin C, and calcium.

SHOPPING LIST

1. Fruits:

- Berries (blueberries, strawberries, raspberries)
- Apples
- Bananas
- Oranges
- Kiwi
- Mango
- Pomegranate

2. Vegetables:

- Spinach
- Kale
- Broccoli
- Bell peppers (assorted colors)
- Carrots
- Zucchini
- Cucumber
- Tomatoes
- Avocado

3. Whole Grains:

- Quinoa
- Brown rice

- Oats (rolled or steel-cut)
- Whole wheat pasta
- Barley

4. Lean Proteins:

- Chicken breast (skinless)
- Turkey breast (ground or whole)
- Salmon
- Cod
- Tofu
- Eggs

5. Legumes:

- Lentils
- Chickpeas
- Black beans
- Kidney beans

6. Dairy and Alternatives:

- Low-fat Greek yogurt
- Low-fat cottage cheese
- Almond milk
- Feta cheese (low-fat)
- Parmesan cheese (grated)

7. Nuts and Seeds:

- Almonds
- Walnuts
- Chia seeds
- Flaxseeds
- Pumpkin seeds

8. Healthy Fats:

- Olive oil (extra virgin)
- Avocado oil
- Coconut oil (for moderation)
- Nut butters (almond, peanut)

9. Herbs and Spices:

- Garlic
- Ginger
- Turmeric
- Basil
- Cilantro
- Rosemary
- Thyme
- Cumin
- Paprika
- Oregano

10. Condiments and Sauces:

- Balsamic vinegar

- Lemon juice
- Low-sodium soy sauce
- Dijon mustard
- Tomato sauce (low-sodium)
- Hummus

11. Whole Grain Products:

- Whole wheat bread
- Whole grain crackers
- Whole grain tortillas

12. Beverages:

- Green tea
- Herbal teas (e.g., chamomile)
- Water

13. Sweeteners:

- Honey
- Maple syrup (for moderation)

14. Frozen Foods:

- Frozen berries
- Frozen vegetables (mixed or individual)

15. Seafood:

- Shrimp
- Mackerel (low in mercury)
- Sardines (packed in water)

16. Miscellaneous:

- Hummus
- Dark chocolate (high cocoa content)
- Dried herbs and spices

17. Dairy Alternatives:

- Soy milk
- Coconut yogurt

18. Grilled Vegetables:

- Eggplant
- Asparagus
- Artichokes

19. Low-Sodium Broth:

- Vegetable broth
- Chicken broth (low-sodium)

20. Fresh Herbs:

- Parsley
- Mint

- Cilantro

CONCLUSION

In conclusion, the AFib diet cookbook for seniors serves as a valuable resource in promoting heart-healthy habits and supporting the well-being of individuals managing atrial fibrillation. By focusing on nutrient-dense, wholesome ingredients and mindful preparation methods, this cookbook aims to provide not just delicious recipes but also a pathway to better cardiovascular health.

The importance of adopting a heart-healthy diet for seniors with AFib cannot be overstated. Through careful food choices, moderation, and an emphasis on key nutrients, individuals can actively contribute to the management of AFib symptoms, reduce potential triggers, and enhance overall cardiovascular function.

As seniors embark on this culinary journey, it is crucial to remember that dietary changes are just one aspect of a comprehensive approach to health. Consulting with healthcare professionals, including cardiologists and registered dietitians, ensures that the dietary recommendations align with individual health needs and contribute to an overall wellness plan.

This cookbook is not just a collection of recipes; it is a tool for empowering seniors to take charge of their health through enjoyable and nourishing meals. It encourages a positive relationship with food, making the journey towards heart-healthy living not only beneficial but also enjoyable.

May these recipes inspire seniors to savor the flavors of nutritious ingredients, explore new culinary horizons, and, most importantly, experience the positive impact of a heart-healthy lifestyle. Here's to good health, delightful meals, and the pursuit of well-being on this flavorful journey with the AFib diet cookbook for seniors.